CYSTIC FIBROSIS

Discoveries, Therapies, and Approaches to Respiratory Health in the Context of Cystic Fibrosis

JACE COOPER

Table of Contents

Introductory 4

CHAPTER ONE 9

Reasons and Heredity...........9

Typical Clinical Presentation
and Symptomatology 13

CHAPTER TWO 20

Therapeutics and
Administration 20

CHAPTER THREE 29

The Experience of CF Daily Life
....29

Disorders and Adverse Events
....36

Conclusion...........................43

THE END................................47

Introductory

Inherited genetic condition that predominantly impacts the respiratory, digestive, and reproductive systems, often known as cystic fibrosis (CF). Mutations in the CFTR gene (cystic fibrosis transmembrane conductance regulator) produce this debilitating and incurable illness. This gene encodes a protein involved in the control of fluid and salt balance throughout the body's cells, particularly those of the lungs and digestive tract.

In people with cystic fibrosis, mucus builds up in the lungs and digestive tract and becomes difficult to expel due to abnormalities in the CFTR gene. It can be difficult to breathe and lead to an increase in respiratory infections if this abnormal mucus blocks airways in the lungs. The thick mucus can obstruct the ducts of the pancreas, preventing the pancreas from releasing enzymes needed to digest food, which can lead to malnutrition and other digestive disorders.

Some of the most frequently encountered signs and symptoms of cystic fibrosis are:

1. Chronic, thick mucus-producing coughing.

2. Inflammation and infection of the lungs occur frequently.

3. Reduced lung capacity and difficulty breathing.

4. Problems digesting and absorbing food lead to stunted development and malnutrition.

5. Skin with a salty flavor.

6. Infertility in males due to obstructed vas deferens.

7. Diabetes and liver disease are more likely to develop.

Airway clearing procedures, medication to thin mucus, antibiotics to cure infections, and nutritional support are all part of the multi-pronged approach to treating cystic fibrosis. In extreme circumstances, a lung transplant may be considered. Despite substantial improvements in life expectancy and quality of life because to medical advancements, CF is still a fatal disease for which there is now no treatment or cure. With proper treatment and care, many people with CF can live into adulthood and beyond.

Families with a history of cystic fibrosis should seek genetic counseling to determine their child's vulnerability to inheriting the disease. Carriers and people at risk of having a child with cystic fibrosis can be identified by prenatal testing and carrier screening.

CHAPTER ONE
Reasons and Heredity

Mutations in the CFTR (cystic fibrosis transmembrane conductance regulator) gene are the most common underlying cause of CF. The protein encoded by this gene is essential for maintaining proper fluid and salt balance inside the body's cells, particularly those of the respiratory and digestive systems. When the CFTR gene is mutated, it can lead to the formation of thick and sticky mucus in many organs, resulting in the distinctive symptoms and problems of CF.

Here are the most important things to know about the genetics and etiology of cystic fibrosis:

1. Cystic fibrosis is inherited in a recessive fashion through one's genes. This indicates that a person needs to receive two defective CFTR gene copies from their parents in order to develop the disease. Carriers (also known as "carriers" or "heterozygotes") inherit one mutant CFTR gene and one normal CFTR gene, but do not often show symptoms of CF. One in four children born to two carriers will develop cystic fibrosis, one in two will be carriers, and one in four will have two normal copies of the CFTR gene.

2. More than 2,000 different mutations in the CFTR gene are known to cause cystic fibrosis. The degree to which these mutations interfere with CFTR function varies. Some mutations result in more severe manifestations of the disease, while others may lead to milder symptoms. The precise combination of mutations an individual has can alter the severity and presentation of the illness.

3. Cystic fibrosis carriers and those at risk of producing a child with the disease can be identified by genetic testing. Couples who have a history of cystic fibrosis in their family, or persons from groups with a higher carrier frequency, are often encouraged to undergo carrier screening. It is also possible to find out if an unborn kid has inherited two mutant CFTR genes through prenatal testing.

4. Mutations in the CFTR gene can sometimes occur without a family history of cystic fibrosis. Individuals without carrier parents may develop cystic fibrosis due to these de novo mutations. These occurrences are quite unusual.

Diagnosis, carrier screening, genetic counseling, and the development of possible treatments and therapies all rely on an understanding of the genetic foundation of cystic fibrosis. Advances in genetic research and therapeutics, such as gene therapy and gene editing, provide hope for improving the lives of individuals with cystic fibrosis by addressing the underlying genetic abnormalities.

Typical Clinical Presentation and Symptomatology

The symptoms of cystic fibrosis (CF) might manifest differently in each individual affected by the disease. The age at which symptoms first appear and how severe they are might also vary. However, cystic fibrosis is characterized by a number of shared symptoms and clinical characteristics.

1. Signs of a Breathing Problem:

• Persistent cough, typically accompanied by thick, sticky mucus, is a common symptom of cystic fibrosis.

Lung infections, such as pneumonia and bronchitis, occur often in people with CF.

Obstructive airway disease and diminished lung function cause wheezing and shortness of breath.

• Lowered exercise tolerance; restricted physical activity because to breathlessness.

• Sputum production: the creation of thick, sticky mucus that is hard to cough up.

2. Signs of Digestion:

• Malnutrition, stunted growth, and vitamin deficiencies may result from difficulties with digestion and absorption of nutrients brought on by cystic fibrosis.

The thick mucus can obstruct the pancreatic ducts, decreasing the production of digestive enzymes and leading to pancreatic insufficiency, which makes digestion difficult.

- Fatty, foul-smelling stools: A classic symptom of malabsorption.

- Pain or discomfort in the abdomen; digestive problems are a common source of this symptom.

3. Differential Diagnosis

Licking the skin or looking for salty residue are both ways to tell whether someone has CF because people with the disease tend to sweat more than average.

Chronic sinusitis and nasal polyps are frequent in CF, leading to congestion in the sinuses and nose.

• Clubbing occurs when the fingers or toes become swollen and rounded.

Women with CF often have limited fertility but can still conceive, whereas men with CF may experience infertility due to a clogged vas deferens.

• Elderly people with CF are at greater risk of developing diabetes because of the disease.

• Cirrhosis and other liver diseases: cystic fibrosis is a known cause of liver illness.

These symptoms can range greatly in both intensity and combination. Some people with CF have modest symptoms, while others have a progressive and debilitating type of the disease. To effectively manage and treat all facets of cystic fibrosis, patients must have access to a multidisciplinary healthcare team that includes pulmonologists, gastroenterologists, nutritionists, and other specialists.

Many people with CF are now able to live active and full lives thanks to the advances in medical treatment and medicines that have made this possible.

CHAPTER TWO
Therapeutics and Administration

The treatment and management of cystic fibrosis (CF) often involve a thorough, multidisciplinary approach focused at treating the many components of the ailment. Treatment for cystic fibrosis focuses on four main areas: pulmonary function, infection management, nutrition, and improving quality of life. Here are the mainstays of care for people with CF:

1. Methods for Cleaning the Airway:

Mucus in the airways can be loosened and cleared with the use of chest physiotherapy techniques like percussion and vibration.

External mechanical vibrations are used by high-frequency chest wall oscillation (HFCWO) devices to help with mucus removal.

Airway clearance can be enhanced with breathing workouts with PEP (positive expiratory pressure) devices.

2. Medications:

• **Mucolytics:** Drugs used to thin mucus, such as dornase alfa (Pulmozyme), so that it can be more easily expelled from the airways.

• Bronchodilators, like albuterol, are drugs that widen the airways and make it easier to breathe.

Antibiotics are used for both curing and avoiding respiratory infections. The medications can be injected, breathed, or ingested.

Airway inflammation can be treated with anti-inflammatory medicines such ibuprofen or corticosteroids.

Some recent drugs improve the function of the CFTR protein by targeting the underlying genetic deficiency in CF; they are called CFTR modulators. Ivacaftor (Kalydeco) and lumacaftor/ivacaftor (Orkambi) are two such medications.

3. Help with Diet:

People with pancreatic insufficiency due to cystic fibrosis may benefit from pancreatic enzyme replacement treatment.

A high-calorie, high-fat diet is commonly recommended to

prevent malnutrition and promote growth.

• Vitamin and mineral supplements: CF can lead to shortages in specific vitamins and minerals, thus supplementation may be recommended.

• Insertion of a gastrostomy (G-) or jejunostomy (J-) tube to allow for direct delivery of nutrients to the stomach or small intestine in cases of severe malnutrition.

4. Rehab for the Lungs:

• Exercise and physical activity: Ongoing physical activity is associated with enhanced pulmonary function, cardiovascular fitness, and general health.

• Breathing techniques, including diaphragmatic and pursed-lip breathing, can be helpful.

5. Containing Infections:

Strict infection control procedures are necessary to prevent the spread of CF between patients.

• Isolation measures may be advised in order to reduce the spread of infectious diseases.

6. Psychological and Emotional Encouragement:

• Individuals and their families can benefit greatly from access to mental health services in order to better manage the effects of CF on daily life.

• Counseling and support groups can be helpful resources for coping with emotional difficulties.

7. Getting a New Set of Lungs:

• Lung transplantation may be explored as a therapy option in severe cases of lung illness.

8. It is crucial to schedule follow-up appointments with a CF care team on a consistent basis in order to track disease development and make any therapy adjustments.

The care team will collaborate closely with the person with CF and their loved ones to develop a unique treatment and management strategy. Many people with CF are now able to live longer, better lives thanks to improvements in medical treatment and CFTR modulator medicines. Individuals with CF should follow their treatment programs and communicate effectively with their healthcare teams to achieve the best possible outcomes.

CHAPTER THREE
The Experience of CF Daily Life

Although having cystic fibrosis (CF) can be difficult, it is possible to live a full and meaningful life with the help of medical treatment and community resources. When managing CF, it's important to keep in mind the following:

1. Management of Health Care:

The importance of sticking to your treatment plan consistently cannot be overstated. Methods of clearing the airway, medication, and scheduled doctor visits all fall under this category.

• Collaborate closely with a wide range of medical professionals, such as gastroenterologists, pulmonologists, nutritionists, respiratory therapists, and social workers.

• Stay up-to-date with prescribed vaccines to prevent respiratory infections.

Tests of pulmonary function should be routinely performed.

2. Food and Nutrition:

To prevent stunting and promote development, it's best to stick to a high-calorie, high-fat diet.

If you have pancreatic insufficiency, you should take pancreatic enzyme supplements.

Remember to drink plenty of water and replenish your salt levels after sweating.

Keep track of your eating habits and weight consistently.

3. If you want better lung capacity, cardiovascular health, and general well-being, then you should exercise often.

• Work out a safe and effective routine with the help of your medical staff.

4. Containing Infections:

• Take proper precautions against spreading germs to other people who suffer from cystic fibrosis.

If your healthcare staff advises you to take isolation measures, make sure you do so.

5. Psychological and Emotional Encouragement:

• Seek out social and psychological aid in coping with CF.

• If you're having emotional or mental health problems, seek out counseling or support groups.

6. Teaching and lobbying:

• Educate yourself thoroughly on cystic fibrosis and its treatment.

Do all you can to help yourself, and use the services and care that are out there?

• If you want to help progress CF treatment, think about taking part in a clinical trial or research study.

7. Changes in Way of Life:

• Juggling CF care with other obligations might be difficult. Effective time management and preparation are crucial.

• Stay away from smoke and other environmental contaminants that may exacerbate breathing difficulties.

Think about how your health and the demands of your job go hand in hand.

8. Transplantation:

• People with CF may occasionally need a lung transplant. If you see a severe reduction in your lung function, talk to your healthcare team about this possibility.

9. Lean on loved ones who will understand and support you.

• Join online and offline CF communities for emotional and practical support.

10. Medication Compliance:

• Proper adherence to treatment programs and the use of recommended drugs are crucial for CF management.

To manage CF symptoms, one must be proactive and well-organized in their healthcare. Life expectancy and quality of life for people with CF have been greatly improved thanks to medical advances including CFTR modulator medicines and enhanced care. Maintaining a positive mindset, close collaboration with a CF care team, and knowledge of the newest advances in CF research and treatment are all crucial. Despite the difficulties associated with CF, a large percentage of people with the disease go on to realize their ambitions, advance in their chosen fields of study or work, and develop satisfying personal relationships.

Disorders and Adverse Events

Many different bodily systems can be negatively impacted by cystic fibrosis (CF) and its related problems. People with CF often have the following problems and related conditions:

1. Problems with Breathing:

Repeated infections with bacteria and viruses such Pseudomonas aeruginosa, Staphylococcus aureus, and Burkholderia cepacia can progressively damage the lungs over time, a condition known as chronic obstructive pulmonary disease (COPD).

Airway damage due to chronic inflammation and mucus buildup is called bronchiectasis. This condition is characterized by the airways enlarging and scarring.

• **Reduced Lung Function**: Over time, lung function may diminish, leading to breathing difficulties and lower exercise tolerance.

• **Respiratory Failure:** CF can lead to respiratory failure in extreme cases, requiring a lung transplant.

2. Problems with the Digestive System:

Poor growth, malnutrition, and malabsorption can result from pancreatic insufficiency, a condition in which the pancreatic ducts get blocked by excess mucus.

- Cirrhosis of the Liver: Liver disease is a known complication of cystic fibrosis.

- Intestinal Obstruction: In some people, excess mucus can build up and cause the intestines to become blocked.

Reduced bile flow can lead to gallstone formation. o Gallstones.

3. Problems with Diet:

- **Malnutrition:** nutritional absorption issues can lead to stunted development.

• **Weight Loss:** It's not uncommon to struggle with keeping the weight at a healthy level.

4. Chronic sinusitis is a common problem for people with cystic fibrosis.

Congestion and trouble breathing through the nose can be caused by nasal polyps.

5.   Complications   with Reproduction and Fertility:

• **Male Infertility:** Men with CF may experience infertility due to a clogged vas deferens.

Women with cystic fibrosis may have diminished fertility, but they are still able to have children.

6. Some people with cystic fibrosis develop diabetes because their bodies have trouble producing insulin and maintaining a healthy glucose balance.

7. Bone Health: Some people with CF develop osteoporosis or low bone density, especially if they are malnourished.

8. Mental Health Issues: Coping with the chronic nature of CF, frequent medical treatments, and potential life-limiting elements of the condition can lead to mental health issues such as anxiety and sadness.

9. Some people with cystic fibrosis experience joint discomfort and inflammation due to a condition called CF-related arthropathy.

10. Joint inflammation and arthritis-like symptoms are also possible complications of cystic fibrosis.

It's worth noting that these consequences can vary in both severity and progression from person to person. The quality of life and longevity of people with CF have been greatly enhanced by medical advances, such as CFTR modulator medicines and enhanced management tactics. These problems and related disorders can be managed and their effects mitigated through consistent monitoring, early intervention, and adherence to treatment strategies. In order to properly address these issues, close cooperation with a healthcare team knowledgeable in CF management is required.

Conclusion

The respiratory and digestive systems are particularly hard hit by cystic fibrosis (CF), a multi-organ hereditary illness. Caused by alterations in the CFTR gene, the disease is characterized by the development of excessive mucus that can cause breathing difficulties, gastrointestinal distress, and other problems. Although CF is a serious and chronic ailment, the quality of life and life expectancy of those who have it have greatly improved thanks to medical improvements.

Managing CF entails a comprehensive, multidisciplinary strategy that includes airway clearance techniques, drugs to address symptoms and underlying genetic problems, nutritional support, infection control measures, and emotional and psychological care. In order to adjust treatment strategies as the condition worsens, close monitoring and consultation with a trained CF care team are required.

Many people with CF go on to have successful and important lives, despite the difficulties brought on by CF. There is optimism for a better prognosis and a cure for cystic fibrosis thanks to ongoing research and medical improvements. When it comes to managing CF and fighting for the best possible results, patients, their families, and their healthcare providers all play an integral role.

THE END